Fizzy World
Of
BATH BOMBS

Amazing Recipes To Create

Beautiful & Creative Bath Bombs

MIRANDA ROSS

TABLE OF CONTENTS

INTRODUCTION

Relaxation and rejuvenation are important keys to a healthy life! When you take out some time to consciously unwind, it fills your day with positivity and light. Since taking bath is a natural step that you do every day, why not add a little zing to it! Your little "me" time will guide you to pamper and indulge yourself a few essential minutes each day and make your skin glow with health and vitality.

Here is when the bath bombs come into the picture! And what pretty stuff they are! They are the balls that when dropped into your bath tub, fizz and create plenty of bubbles which ensconces you into a luxurious spa-like ambience! Add some soothing music and voila, you get the perfect setting for a date with yourself!

This book is a guide to understanding more on bath bombs, its numerous benefits and ways of use. It is a guide to help you get started with creating your own colorful, attractive and heavenly bath bombs. They are pretty inexpensive and amazing self-care items which you can begin at home. You will also find some extremely useful tips and advises on questions regarding the bath bombs.

This book also has some simple, yet blissful recipes of bath bombs that you can make. There are different bath bombs with ingredients like herbs, essential oils, etc., that will help you relax, rejuvenate and indulge yourself. No matter what your mood is, there would be a bath bomb to compliment it!

It is time to create some bombs that are cost efficient and bring peace and tranquility to your mind. Let's begin. Let's dive in!

This document is geared towards providing exact and reliable information in regards to the topic and issue covered. The publication is sold with the idea that the publisher is not required to render accounting, officially permitted, or otherwise, qualified services. If advice is necessary, legal or professional, a practiced individual in the profession should be ordered.

From a Declaration of Principles which was accepted and approved equally by a Committee of the American Bar Association and a Committee of Publishers and Associations.

The information provided herein is stated to be truthful and consistent, in that any liability, in terms of inattention or otherwise, by any usage or abuse of any policies, processes, or directions contained within is the solitary and utter responsibility of the recipient reader. Under no circumstances will any legal responsibility or blame be held against the publisher for any reparation, damages, or monetary loss due to the information herein, either directly or indirectly.

The information herein is offered for informational purposes solely, and is universal as so. The presentation of the information is without contract or any type of guarantee assurance.

The trademarks that are used are without any consent, and the publication of the trademark is without permission or backing by the trademark owner. All trademarks and brands within this book are for clarifying purposes only and are the owned by the owners themselves, not affiliated with this document.

DISCLAIMER: The purpose of this book is to provide information only. The information, though believed to be entirely accurate, is NOT a substitution for medical, psychological or professional advice, diagnosis or treatment. The author recommends that you seek the advice of your physician or other qualified health care provider to present them with questions you may have regarding any medical condition. Advice from your trusted, professional medical advisor should always supersede information presented in this book.

THE BEAUTY OF BATH BOMBS
BENEFITS AND USES

Bath bombs! The name sounds very quirky yet helps you visualize what the bomb may do to your bath. Nothing brings more happiness than a dip in a hot bath to pamper yourself. You can make it ritualistic by tossing in a bomb! The bombs are dry and packed with citric acid and baking soda. When they are dry, they are fairly unreactive, however, once they touch water, they react strongly to create a characteristic fizzing that lasts for a few minutes. The carbon dioxide that is released is nice, ticklish and quite pleasurable. The other ingredients in the bomb such as essential oils, butter and herbs impart a great feel and fragrance that relaxes you. It enhances the entire experience of taking a bath!

Bath bombs can be created by both the novice and the experts. You can make them in all shapes, colors, and sizes. The process of creating these luxuries are simple, but it definitely takes practice. Since the bath bombs are very sensitive to moisture, extra care needs to be taken to create them and in the right composition so that they don't crumble, drown or fall apart without fizzing as they should.

So why not try your hand at making some perfect beauties, to bring you the goodness and vitality when you take your simple bath?

THE BENEFITS OF BATH BOMBS

- The bath bombs come with many moisturizing and skin-nourishing oils and butter that make your skin supple and alive. They work wonders on dry skin.
- Essential oils like lavender and chamomile not once improve the smell of the bath, but also help you feel relaxed and awake.
- Additive like dried flowers and glitter may float on the top and serves as a great esthetic goal.
- Salts and powdered clay also help to nourish and moisturize your skin.

USES OF BATH BOMBS

- There are many uses of bath bombs, the primary one being the feeling of being pampered and indulged. You feel relaxed after a few minutes in such an environment. Create a spa-like atmosphere. Add music, take a book and soak in. Or have something hot to drink or just wear a face mask. By the time you finish the bath, your mask would do its job and help you look great.

- Bath bombs that have essential oils like eucalyptus oil help you with sinus relief. Just use warm water in the tub and drop in a bomb and relax. Other bath bombs with specific essential oils help you relieve muscle pain and improve sleep.

- Use bath bombs for aromatherapy, which will make you feel less stressed and more awake. It will reduce anxiety and lift depression and leave you energized and lively. Hence, choose the bath bombs accordingly.

- You can also display a bath bomb in a nice cool dish in the bathroom. It will disintegrate slowly and act as an air freshener with a nice subtle fragrance.

BATH BOMBS

USEFUL TIPS AND ADVISES

Bath bombs are a delightful way to enjoy and slow down for some time. They are simple and quite easy to make, however, any small strange reason can prompt your bombs to go weird. Things like the room temperature, humidity, inconsistent in portions of ingredients, etc. can trigger the doom of the bombs. Let me give you some basic and useful tips that will help you create superb bombs and divert disasters.

THE SHOPPING LIST TO MAKE IT EASY

To have a smooth and productive experience, here are a few things that you need to buy.

1. Baking Soda: The best would be the fine food-grade Sodium Bicarbonate. Other technical grades may have granules and impurities that may not give the best results.

2. Citric Acid: The best here would be fine grained or table salt sized. Powdered ones may be too volatile and granules don't work that well. Get the best from the supermarket, spice shops or wine making suppliers.

3. Cornstarch: This is needed to control the fizzing reaction that takes place between the ingredients as you mix them.

4. Witch Hazel: It is sometimes better to use witch hazel instead of water. This helps your bath bombs to dry sooner and thus allows you to remove them from their molds faster. Also, water tends to set off the ingredients in the bath bombs before time, hence you may exchange it with witch hazel.

5. Essential oils: You can buy the from food stores or online and use them in small amounts. However, sometimes essential oils can dull or enhance effects of drugs. So, if you have any medical condition or are pregnant, use them after consulting the doctor. Also, before using any oil, dilute oil and do a skin patch irritation test before using them. Also when you buy fragrance oils, make sure they are body safe and not used for candle making etc.

6. Food Colors: Get the colors of your choice. Also, make sure you don't overuse it, as it might stain the bath tub if used liberally.

7. Spritzer bottle

8. Rubber Gloves: It is best to use one while mixing the ingredients since citric acid tends to cause skin irritation and also remove your nail paint!

9. Glass Bowl/Plastic Mixing Bowl: Opt for glass ones as often as possible as they are non-reactive.

10. Mold: Now get creative and get a variety so you have different shapes of divine bath bomb pleasures.

11. Optional Ingredients: Vegetable oils, Mineral salts, Sea salts etc.

STORAGE AND OTHER TIPS

1. The golden rule is to store the bath bombs into airtight containers like Tupperware at room temperature only after the bombs are completely dry. If they are even a little moist, they will crumble down.

2. Store the different scents and flavors separately since the scents would otherwise combine with one another with time.

3. Use the bath bombs within 6 months. The quality will degrade after that.

4. To extend the life of plastic molds, remove the bath bombs once they dry and wash the molds thoroughly and immediately.

5. Be sure to check if you are allergic to anything before including it to your bath both. If you have sensitive skin, be cautious. If you are allergic to bubble baths and bath oils, you may be allergic to bath bombs.

FREQUENTLY FACED QUESTIONS

What is the reason for the cracking, crumbling bombs?

If the bomb crumbles, it means the mixture may be too dry. You may add a spritz of witch hazel or essential oils to moisten them which helps them to stay together once they dry. Also, make sure they are not too wet otherwise they might crumble after you place them in the mold. The right amount of moisture is the key to firm a beautiful bomb.

What is the reason for the bombs not fizzing as they should?

Sometimes you find your bombs fizzing weakly in the bathtub, and if it does, try to increase the amount of citric acid in your recipe. So 2 parts of baking soda and 1.5 parts of citric acid. However, if you are using cornstarch, decrease the amount of citric acid. Fizzing is also affected if you use a large amount of oil. Fizzing also decreases if you leave the bombs in the open and it attracts moisture from the environment. Always wrap the bomb with a plastic wrap to protect it.

What is the reason for a soft bomb and a clumpy bomb?

If the bomb is soft, it may contain excess moisture. Be care when you add witch hazel or water and compensate with dry ingredients if you mistakenly add more liquid. You may also add cornstarch or clay if you wish to have sturdy bombs. Also, when you mix the ingredients, mix well or they would clump. So before you add oil or water, just remove the clumps with your fingers and make them as smooth as possible. You may also use a mesh sifter to remove the clumps and get a fine mixture. Also after mixing oil, make sure you work hard to mix it thoroughly.

How many colors can you use?

Since baking soda and citric acid are white, you may need to use some color or a lot of it to get your desired hue. However, remember, a lot of color may stain your skin and the bathtub. You can use the various food colors or the color available in the market, especially for the bath bombs.

What are the best molds for bath bombs?

There are many two part molds that are great for bombs. Molds can be sturdy yet slightly inflexible. You can use plastic mold, silicone molds or heavy duty molds. To get a well-made bomb, leave the mixture to dry in the mold overnight or even a day or two. If you remove it earlier, it may crumble.

What is the correct way to package a bomb?

Bath bombs are very delicate. They need to be packaged with care. You can use airtight boxes, jars, and bags. You may also use molds that can keep the bombs safe till use. If you live in a humid place, wrap the bombs in plastic wraps and then keep them in airtight jars. You can also keep a silica packet along with the bombs so that it absorbs the excess moisture.

What is the life span of a bomb?

Bath bombs are good for 6 months. If you wait longer, the bomb may lose its amazing fizzing power and become weak. Though baking soda and citric acid, both have a long shelf life, citric acid can lose its potency. However, its strength remains, if it is kept in airtight containers. Yet, to be safe, use them within the time span. After all there may be different shelf lives for the other ingredients in the bomb.

Bath bombs make perfect gifts for yourself and your friends. Age and occasions don't matter. You can gift them for birthdays, baby showers, weddings or just as "thank-you" gifts. You can also make these homemade safe products for selling. Many people would love to buy such beautiful and gorgeous products.

Bomb Recipes
FOR COMPLETE ENERGIZATION AND RELAXATION

Recipe # 1
The Tangy Ocean Breeze Bath Bomb

Ingredients:

2 cups baking soda

¼ cup Epsom salt

¼ cup cornstarch

1 cup citric acid (powdered)

1 tsp. sea salt

1 tbsp. sweet almond oil

10 drops ocean breeze/rain fragrance oil

Spritzer of witch hazel/water

Instructions:

1. Place the baking powder, citric acid, Epsom salt and cornstarch in a mixing bowl and blend them thoroughly.
2. Add the fragrance oil to the sweet almond oil and add them to the mixture. Stir well.

3. Add a spritz or two of water or witch hazel to the mixture and make a consistent mix.

4. Press the mixture into the bomb mold of your choice and let them dry in a cool, dry place.

5. Once completely dry, remove the bombs gently and store them into an airtight container.

Recipe # 2
Energizing Passion Bath Bomb

Ingredients:

2 cups baking soda

2 tbsp. cornstarch

1 cup citric acid (powdered)

¼ cup Epsom salt

1 tbsp. sweet almond oil

4 drops mandarin essential oil

4 drops sandalwood essential oil

4 drops jasmine essential oil

Spritzer of witch hazel/water

Instructions:

1. Place the baking soda, citric acid, corn starch and Epsom salt in a bowl and mix them thoroughly.
2. Add the essential oils into the sweet almond oil and add them to the mixture. Stir well.
3. Add a spritz or two of water or witch hazel and moisten the mixture so that when you knead the mix, it can take a shape of a ball without crumbling.
4. Pack the mixture tightly into molds and keep them aside for a day or two to dry.

5. Once the bombs are completely dry, remove them gently and store them in airtight containers.

Recipe # 3
Ultimate Relaxation Bath Bomb

Ingredients:

2 cups baking soda

¼ cup Epsom salt

¼ cup cornstarch

1 cup citric acid (powdered)

1 tbsp. sweet almond oil

4 drops geranium essential oil

4 drops sandalwood essential oil

4 drops lavender essential oil

Spritzer of witch hazel/water

Instructions:

1. Place the baking soda, cornstarch, citric acid and Epsom salt in a bowl and mix them well.
2. Add the essential oil to the sweet almond oil and then add the oil to the mixture. Stir well.
3. Add a spritz or two of water or witch hazel and moisten the mixture to get a consistent mix that looks like wet sand.
4. Pack the mixture into the molds tightly.
5. Keep the molds aside for a day or two to dry completely.

6. Once they dry off, gently remove the bombs from the molds and store them in airtight containers.

Recipe # 4
Fresh Forest Bath Bomb

Ingredients:

2 cups baking soda

¼ cup Epsom salt

¼ cup cornstarch

1 cup citric acid (powdered)

1 tbsp. sweet almond oil

10 drops cedar wood atlas oil

Spritzer of witch hazel/water

Instructions:

1. Place the dry ingredients like baking soda, cornstarch, citric acid and Epsom salt in a bowl and mix them well.
2. Add the essential oil to the sweet almond oil and then add the oil to the mixture. Stir well.
3. Add a spritz or two of water or witch hazel and moisten the mixture so that when you knead the mix, it can take a shape of a ball without crumbling.
4. Pack the mixture into the molds tightly.
5. Keep the molds aside for a day or two to dry completely.

6. Once they dry off, gently remove the bombs from the molds and store them in airtight containers.

Recipe # 5
Refreshing Ginger Bath Bomb

Ingredients:

¼ cups baking soda

¼ cup citric acid (powdered)

6 tbsp. Shea butter

½ cup cornstarch

3 tbsp. almond oil

3 tbsp. coconut oil

1 tsp. ginger essential oil

Spritzer of witch hazel/water

Red and yellow food coloring (optional)

Instructions:

1. Mix the baking soda, citric acid and cornstarch in a bowl.
2. Add the Shea butter and coconut oil to the bowl and mix well.
3. Add the almond oil and the ginger essential oil and stir consistently.
4. Then add the red and yellow food coloring now to get the color of your choice.

5. Add a spritz or two of water or witch hazel and moisten the mixture to get the desired wet sand consistency.
6. Press this consistent mix into the molds tightly.
7. Keep the molds aside for a day or two to dry completely.
8. Once they dry off, gently remove the bombs from the molds and store them in airtight containers for later use.

Bomb Recipes
WITH HERBS

Recipe # 1
Fresh Minty Bath Bomb

Ingredients:

2 cups baking soda

¼ cup Epsom salt

¼ cup cornstarch

1 cup citric acid (powdered)

1 tbsp. extra virgin coconut oil

10 drops peppermint essential oil

Spritzer of witch hazel/water

Fresh mint sprigs

Instructions:

1. Place the baking soda, cornstarch, citric acid and Epsom salt and mix them thoroughly.
2. Melt the coconut oil gently and the peppermint oil to it. Add the oil to the mixture.
3. Add a spritz or two of water or witch hazel and moisten the mixture so that when you knead the mix, it can take a shape of a ball without crumbling.

4. Add a sprig of mint to the bottom of the mold and pack the mix in the molds tightly.

5. Keep the molds aside to dry completely.

6. Once they dry off, gently remove them from molds and store them in airtight containers.

Recipe # 2
Green Tea Bath Bomb

Ingredients:

2 cups baking soda

¼ cup Epsom salt

¼ cup cornstarch

1 cup citric acid (powdered)

3 tbsp. strong green tea

1 tbsp. dried green tea leaves (crumbled)

Spritzer of witch hazel/water

Instructions:

1. Place the baking soda, cornstarch, citric acid and Epsom salt in a bowl and mix them thoroughly.
2. Brew a strong cup of green tea. Take 3 tablespoons of it and add them to the dry mixture. Add the tea slowly, bit by bit, so that the baking soda and citric acid do not go off.
3. Add the crumbled dry green leaves to the mixture as well.
4. Add a spritz or two of water or witch hazel and moisten the mixture to get the required consistency.
5. Pack the mixture into the molds tightly and keep the molds aside for a day or two to dry completely.

6. Once they dry off, gently remove the bomb from the molds and store them in airtight containers.

Recipe # 3
Dried Flowers Bath Bomb

Ingredients:

2 cups baking soda

3 tsp. olive oil

1 cup cornstarch

1 cup citric acid

5 drops food coloring

1 tsp. lavender essential oil

Dried flowers

Spritzer of witch hazel/water

Instructions:

1. Mix the dry ingredients like the baking powder, cornstarch, and citric acid as well as the dried flowers.
2. Mix the oil and add this to this mixture. Stir well. Add food coloring of your choice.
3. Add a spritz or two of water or witch hazel and moisten the mixture to get the required consistency.
4. Place them into mold tightly and let them dry well.
5. Store in airtight container for future use.

Recipe # 4
Coconut and Lime Bath Bomb

Ingredients:

1 cup baking soda

½ cup citric acid

1 cup cornstarch

1 cup rice bran powder

1 cup coconut milk powder

¾ cup brown sugar

1 tbsp. cocoa powder

2 oz. mango butter

3 oz. organic virgin coconut cream oil

5 tsp. lime essential oil

A bit of lime zest

Spritzer of witch hazel/water

Instructions:

1. Mix the dry ingredients like the baking powder, citric acid, cornstarch, coconut milk powder, rice bran powder, sugar, lime zest and cocoa powder.
2. Mix the butter and oil and add them to this mixture. Stir well.

3. Add a spritz or two of water or witch hazel and moisten the mixture so that when you knead the mix, it can take a shape of a ball without crumbling.

4. Place them into mold tightly and let them dry well.

5. Store in airtight container for future use.

Recipe # 5
Lemongrass Lavender Bath Bomb

Ingredients:

1 cup baking soda

½ cup citric acid

1 cup cornstarch

5 tsp. lemongrass essential oil

Dried lavender herbs

Spritzer of witch hazel/water

Instructions:

1. Place the baking soda, cornstarch, citric acid and the dried lavender herbs and mix them thoroughly.
2. Add the lemongrass essential oil to the mixture.
3. Add a spritz or two of water or witch hazel and moisten the mixture.
4. Add a few dried herbs to the bottom of the mold and pack the mix in the molds tightly.
5. Keep the molds aside to dry completely.
6. Once they dry off, gently remove them from molds and store them in airtight containers.

Bomb Recipes
WITH ESSENTIAL OILS AND BUTTER

Recipe # 1
Moisturizing Cocoa Butter Bath Bombs

Ingredients:

2 cups baking soda

¼ cup Epsom salt

1 cup citric acid (powdered)

¼ cup cornstarch

1 tbsp. cocoa powder

1 tbsp. coconut oil

Spritzer of witch hazel/water

Instructions:

1. Add the baking soda, cornstarch, citric acid and Epsom salt and mix them thoroughly.
2. Melt the coconut oil and then add the oil to the mix, stirring constantly.
3. Spritz water or witch hazel to the mixture to moisten and then make a ball using your hands and place them into molds.

4. Place the cocoa powder in a thin layer in the mold. Pack the mold tightly and let it dry for a day or two so that they are completely dry.

5. Store in an airtight dry space until further use.

Recipe # 2
Vanilla Cocoa Cream Bath Bomb

Ingredients:

2 cups baking soda

¼ cup Epsom salt

1 cup citric acid (powdered)

¼ cup cornstarch

1 tsp. white rock crystal sugar

A few drops of vanilla

1 tbsp. cocoa powder

1 tbsp. cocoa butter

1 tbsp. extra virgin coconut oil

Spritzer of witch hazel/water

Instructions:

1. Place the baking soda, cornstarch, citric acid and Epsom salt and make sure they are mixed thoroughly.
2. Melt the coconut oil and cocoa butter gently and add them to the mix. Also, add the drops of vanilla and mix thoroughly.
3. Use a spritz or two of water or witch hazel and make it moist like wet sand. Then using your hands, place them in molds of your choice and layer the cocoa powder and pack the molds tightly.

4. Leave them to dry for a day or two and then store in a dry airtight container until use.

Recipe # 3
Orange Cream Bath Bomb

Ingredients:

2 cups baking soda

¼ cup Epsom salt

¼ cup cornstarch

1 cup citric acid (powdered)

2 tbsp. soy milk powder

1 tbsp. sweet almond oil

6 drops bergamot essential oil

6 drops orange essential oil

Spritzer of witch hazel/water

Natural orange clay for color (optional)

Instructions:

1. Place the baking soda, cornstarch, citric acid, soy milk powder and Epsom salt and make sure they are mixed thoroughly. You may add orange clay to the mix to get the orange color.
2. Add the essential oils to the almond oil and gently add them to the mix. Blend thoroughly.
3. You may use a spritz or two of water or witch hazel to moisten the mixture to get a consistent blend.

4. Leave the molds till they dry off completely (a day or two) and then store them in the airtight containers until future use.

Recipe # 4
Tri-Butter Bath Bomb

Ingredients:

2 cups baking soda

¼ cup Epsom salt

¼ cup cornstarch

1 cup citric acid (powdered)

1 tbsp. cocoa butter

1 tsp. avocado butter

1 tsp. aloe vera butter

10 drops lavender essential oil

Spritzer of witch hazel/water

Instructions:

1. Place the baking soda, citric acid, Epsom salt and cornstarch in a bowl and mix them thoroughly.
2. Gently melt the three types of butter and add the drops of lavender essential oil into it.
3. Add this to the mixture and stir them.
4. Add a spritz or two of water or witch hazel to moisten the mix so that when you knead the mix, it holds the shape of a ball.
5. Place the bombs in the molds and pack the molds tightly.

6. Let the molds dry for a day or two in a cool dry place and then store them into airtight containers.

Recipe # 5
Anise-Shea Butter Bath Bomb

Ingredients:

2 cups baking soda

¼ cup Epsom salt

¼ cup cornstarch

1 cup citric acid (powdered)

1 tbsp. Shea butter

Dried anise pods (whole stars)

10 drops star anise essential oil

Spritzer of witch hazel/water

Instructions:

1. Place the baking soda, citric acid, Epsom salt and cornstarch in a bowl and mix them thoroughly.
2. Melt the Shea butter gently and add the anise oil to it and mix it to the other ingredients.
3. Add a spritz or two of water or witch hazel and moisten the entire mixture so that it looks like wet sand.
4. Knead the mix into a ball. Then add a dried anise star pod into the bottom of each mold and pack the mix tightly into the mold. Let the mix dry off completely.

5. Gently remove the bombs from the mold and store them into the airtight containers for future use.

Bomb Recipes
WITH CITRUSY FLAVOR

Recipe # 1:
Fresh Lemon Bath Bomb

Ingredients:

1 cup baking soda

¾ cup cornstarch

½ cup citric acid (powdered)

1 ½ tsp. lemon eucalyptus essential oil

1 tsp. spearmint essential oil

Spritzer of witch hazel/water

Instructions:

1. Place the baking soda, cornstarch, and citric acid in a bowl and mix thoroughly so there are no clumps.
2. Slowing pour in the essential oils into the mix and stir them often.
3. Mix thoroughly and then add in a spritz or two of water or witch hazel to moisten the mixture. Stir the ingredients so that they don't react. Once they are like wet sand, place them on molds of your choice and leave them overnight to dry.

4. Once dry, remove the lemony bombs carefully and store them in airtight containers until you wish to use them.

Recipe # 2
Sweet Mandarin Orange Bath Bomb

Ingredients:

1 cup baking soda

½ cup citric acid (powdered)

¾ cup cornstarch

2 tsp. mandarin orange essential oil

Spritzer of witch hazel/water

Red and yellow food colors (optional)

Instructions:

1. Combine and mix the baking soda, cornstarch, and the citric acid in a bowl.

2. Slowly add the mandarin orange essential oil to the mix and pause and mix. You may also add the red and yellow food color to the mix and stir well to get the fresh orange color.

3. Press this mix into the molds of your choice. If the mixture is too dry, add a spritz of water or witch hazel. Let the mixture dry completely overnight in the molds.

4. Once it's dry, remove from molds and store in airtight container for later use.

Recipe # 3
Zingy Grapefruit Bath Bomb

Ingredients:

1 cup baking soda

½ cup citric acid (powdered)

¾ cup cornstarch

2 tsp. grapefruit essential oil

Spritzer of witch hazel/water

Red and yellow food colors (optional)

Instructions:

1. Mix the baking soda, citric acid and cornstarch in a bowl and mix thoroughly.

2. Pour in the essential oil slowly and keep stirring the mixture.

3. You may also add the food coloring to get a grapefruit-like color. Take 3 drops of red and 2 drops of yellow color and mix thoroughly.

4. Add a spritz or two of water or witch hazel to moisten the mix like wet sand.

5. Place the mix in the mold with steady hands and let it completely dry off.

6. Remove them carefully from the molds and store in airtight containers until use.

Recipe # 4
Spicy Orange Bath Bomb

Ingredients:

1 cup baking soda

½ cup citric acid (powdered)

¾ cup cornstarch

1 tsp. bitter orange essential oil

1 tsp. nutmeg essential oil

1 tsp. cardamom essential oil

Spritzer of witch hazel/water

Red, green and yellow food colors (optional)

Instructions:

1. Mix the baking soda, citric acid and cornstarch in a bowl and mix thoroughly.
2. Pour in the essential oils slowly and keep stirring the mixture.
3. You may also add the food coloring to get an orange and nutmeg brown like color.
4. Give a spritz or two of water or witch hazel to moisten the mix like wet sand so that when you knead the mix, it can take a shape of a ball without crumbling.
5. Place the mix in the mold with steady hands and let it completely dry off.

6. Remove them carefully from the molds and store in airtight containers until use.

Recipe # 5:
Lime 'n' Lemony Bath Bomb

Ingredients:

1 cup baking soda

½ cup citric acid (powdered)

¾ cup cornstarch

1 tsp. almond oil

1 tsp. lemon essential oil

1 tsp. lime essential oil

Zest of lime and lemon

Green and yellow food coloring

Spritzer of witch hazel/water

Plastic snap-together mold

Instructions:

1. Mix the baking soda, citric acid and cornstarch in a bowl and mix thoroughly.

2. Pour in the essential oils and almond oil slowly and keep stirring the mixture. Add the zest of lime and lemon to the mix.

3. Separate the mixture into two bowls. Add drops of green color to one bowl and yellow color to other.

4. Give a spritz or two of water or witch hazel to moisten them, so that they look like wet sand and don't crumble when you make a ball of them.

5. Place the mix in the snap-together mold with green on one side and yellow on the other. Snap them together with steady hand and let it completely dry off.

6. Remove them carefully and store in airtight containers until use.

Bomb Recipes
FOR BETTER HEALTH

Recipe # 1
Bath Bomb for Cold and Flu Relief

Ingredients:

2 cups baking soda

¼ cup cornstarch

¼ cup Epsom salt

1 tbsp. sweet almond oil

1 cup citric acid (powdered)

6 drops eucalyptus essential oil

6 drops chamomile essential oil

6 drops peppermint essential oil

Spritzer of witch hazel/water

Instructions:

1. Mix the baking soda, cornstarch, citric acid and Epsom salt and mix them thoroughly. Add the essential oils and sweet almond oil and blend them in.
2. You may use a spritz or two of water or witch hazel to get the correct texture of the mixture.

3. Place the mixture into the molds and let them dry completely.
4. Once they are dry remove them carefully from the molds and store them in an airtight container for future use.

Recipe # 2
Bath Bomb for Muscle and Joint Pain Relief

Ingredients:

2 cups baking soda

¼ cup cornstarch

1 cup citric acid (powdered)

¼ cup Epsom salt

1 tbsp. coconut oil

5 drops black pepper oil

10 drops lemon essential oil

Spritzer of witch hazel/water

Instructions:

1. Combine baking soda, citric acid, cornstarch and Epsom salt and mix them thoroughly. Add the melted coconut oil and other essential oils to the mixture.

2. You may use a spritz or two of water or witch hazel to get the correct texture of the mix.

3. Place the mixture into the molds and let them dry completely.

4. Once they are dry remove them carefully from the molds and store them in an airtight container for future use.

Recipe # 3
Bath Bomb for Inducing Better Sleep

Ingredients:

2 cups baking soda

¼ cup cornstarch

1 cup citric acid (powdered)

¼ cup Epsom salt

2 ½ tbsp. grapeseed oil

4 drops lavender essential oil

4 drops tangerine essential oil

4 drops ylang-ylang essential oil

4 drops marjoram oil

4 drops orange essential oil

Liquid food color for hue of your choice

Spritzer of witch hazel/water

Instructions:

1. Combine baking soda, citric acid, cornstarch and Epsom salt and mix them thoroughly.
2. Add all the oils to the mix and blend them. Add food color of your choice.
3. You may use a spritz or two of water or witch hazel to get the correct texture of the mix.

4. Place the mixture into the molds and let them dry completely.

5. Once they are dry remove them carefully from the molds and store them in an airtight container for future use.

Bomb Recipes
FOR THE PERFECT
"GIFT-BOMBS"

Recipe # 1
Valentine's Day Bath Bomb

Ingredients:

1 cup baking soda

½ cup citric acid (powdered)

¼ cup cane sugar

¾ cup cornstarch

2 tbsp. jasmine essential oil

Red food coloring or/and dried ground strawberries and blackberries

Spritzer of witch hazel/water

Instructions:

1. Mix the baking soda, citric acid, cane sugar and cornstarch in a bowl. If you find dried berries, add them to the mix and stir well.

2. Slowly add the essential oil to the mixture while stirring and then a few drops of red food color, if you have them.

3. Add a spritz or two of water or witch hazel and moisten the mixture for the correct consistency.
4. It would work great if you have heart shaped molds or use a heart cookie cutter.
5. Pack the mixture into the molds tightly and keep the molds aside to dry off completely.
6. Once they dry off after a day or two, gently remove the bomb from the molds and store them in airtight containers and use them for your steamy bubble bath.

Recipe # 2
Yummy Cake Bath Bomb

Ingredients:

1 cup baking soda

½ cup citric acid (powdered)

2 tbsp. cocoa butter

¼ cup Epsom salt

¼ cup cornstarch

1 tsp. almond oil

1 tsp. vanilla essential oil

Yellow food coloring

Cupcake liners and cupcake/muffin tins

Spritzer of witch hazel/water

Ingredients for the icing:

1 ½ cup powdered sugar

2 ½ tbsp. meringue powder

4 tbsp. warm distilled water

¼ tsp. cream of tartar

½ tsp. vanilla essential oil

Piping bag and nozzles

Instructions:

1. Place the baking soda, citric acid, Epsom salt and cornstarch in a bowl and mix thoroughly. Add the cocoa butter and mix well.
2. Add the essential oils slowly and stir frequently. Add a drop or two of yellow food coloring to the mix.
3. Add a spritz or two of water or witch hazel and moisten the mixture.
4. Fill the cupcake tins with liners and then press the mix into the tins and let them dry for 4-6 hours.

For Icing:

1. Mix the meringue powder and the water in a bowl. Then add cream of tartar to the mix and stir.
2. Then add the powdered sugar and whisk the mix with an electric whisk until you get a frothy mix that stays in shape. Then add the essential oil to the mix.
3. Quickly move the mix into a piping bag and give an icing to the cake bombs. Once done, leave them to set for another 24 hours and store them into airtight containers.
4. They sure make lovely gifts!

Recipe # 3
Disco Party Bath Bomb

Ingredients:

1 cup baking soda

½ cup citric acid (powdered)

¾ cup cornstarch

1 tsp. almond oil

1 tsp. star anise essential oil

1 tsp. cosmetic glitter

1 tsp. edible glitter (don't use craft glitter)

Blue food coloring

Plastic Christmas snap together ornaments

Spritzer of witch hazel/water

Instructions:

1. Mix the baking soda, citric acid and cornstarch in a bowl and mix well. Add the almond oil and star anise oil to the mix and stir well.

2. Now add the cosmetic glitter and half of the edible glitter.

3. Add a drop of blue coloring to get a light blue tint. You may use a spritz of water or witch hazel to get the correct texture of the mixture.

4. At the bottom of the snap together ornament, add some edible glitter and then pack the bomb mixture firmly into the molds and close the halves together and leave them to dry.

5. Wait for a day or two and remove them gently from the molds. Place them in airtight containers till later use.

Recipe # 4
Winter Snowball Bath Bomb

Ingredients:

½ cup baking soda

¼ cup Epsom Salt

¼ cup cornstarch

2 ½ tsp. almond oil

¼ cup citric acid (powdered)

4 drops fir needle essential oil

4 drops spearmint essential oil

Blue food coloring

Spritzer of witch hazel/water

Instructions:

1. Mix together the baking soda, cornstarch, Epsom salt and citric acid in a bowl thoroughly.

2. Gradually add the almond oil and the essential oils to the mixture and stir well. Add the blue coloring to get the hue of your choice.

3. You may use a spritz or two of water or witch hazel to get the correct texture of the mixture.

4. Press the mix firmly into round molds or an ice-cream scoop.

5. Leave the mix to dry completely and then remove carefully from the molds.
6. Store them in airtight containers and gift them with pleasure.

Recipe # 5
Christmassy Bath Bomb

Ingredients:

1 cup baking soda

½ cup citric acid (powdered)

¾ cup cornstarch

1 tsp. Myrrh essential oil

1 tsp. Frankincense essential oil

Red and green food coloring

Spritzer of witch hazel/water

Plastic ornaments snap together ornaments

Instructions:

1. Mix together the baking soda, cornstarch, and citric acid in a bowl thoroughly.
2. Gradually add the essential oils to the mixture and stir well.
3. Now separate the mixture in two halves and place them in two separate bowls.
4. Add a few drops of red food color to one bowl and mix thoroughly and add drops of green food color to the other bowl and do likewise.
5. You may use a spritz or two of water or witch hazel to get the correct composition of the mixture.

6. For the Christmassy look, press the red mix firmly into one part of the mold and the green mix to the other half of the mold. Snap the parts together so that there are both red and green parts in the bath bomb. Try different combinations of red and green by layering or using different ways to create news designs.

7. Leave the mix to dry completely and then remove carefully from the molds.

8. Store them in airtight containers and use them later as awesome gifts.

Recipe # 6
Fortune Cookie Bath Bomb

Ingredients:

2 cups baking soda

½ cup cornstarch

1 cup citric acid (powdered)

¼ cup Epsom salt

¼ cup milk powder

2 tbsp. cocoa butter (softened)

2 tbsp. almond oil

1 tsp. Bergamot essential oil

1 tsp. lavender essential oil

Yellow food coloring

Spritzer of witch hazel/water

Fortune cookie soap mold

Laminated fortune slips printed

Instructions:

1. Mix the dry ingredients like the cornstarch, citric acid, baking soda and milk powder in a glass bowl thoroughly.
2. Add the essential oils to the almond oil and cocoa butter and then add them to the dry mixture and mix well.

3. Add the yellow color to get the hue of your choice and stir well.

4. You may use a spritz or two of water or witch hazel to get the right composition of the mixture.

5. To make an authentic fortune cookie bomb, press the mixture firmly till half of the fortune cookie mold and then add the laminated fortune slip and cover with the rest of the mix.

6. Leave the mix to dry completely and then remove carefully from the molds.

7. Store them in airtight containers and use them later as amazing gifts.

Recipe # 7
Golden Glow Bath Bomb

Ingredients:

2 cup baking soda

1 cup citric acid (powdered)

4 ml orange grove fragrance oil

4 ml champagne fragrance oil

2 tbsp. meadow foam oil

2 tbsp. cocoa butter (softened)

King's Gold Mica

Coral orange la bomb

Spritzer of witch hazel/water

99% Isopropyl Alcohol (rubbing alcohol)

Instructions:

1. In a mixing bowl, add the citric acid, baking powder, and mix well.
2. Add the oils with cocoa butter and add them to the mixture. Keep on stirring.
3. Add a few drops of the coral orange la bomb and mix thoroughly to get the color of your choice.
4. You may use a spritz or two of water or witch hazel to get the appropriate texture of the mixture.

5. Place the mixture into the molds and let them dry completely.

6. Once they are dry remove them carefully from the molds.

7. In a bowl, place the king's gold mica. Use a spritzer and spritz 99% isopropyl alcohol on the outside of a bomb and then gently roll the bomb in the gold mica in the bowl. Use the fingers to remove excess mica. Then make sure they are completely dry before you store them in an airtight container or place them back in same molds as before until later use.

8. They look visually stunning and leave a gold shimmer on your body!

CONCLUSION

Bath bombs not only look amazingly great, they also are a regal and fun way to unwind and relax. With the ingredients that include butter and essential oils, bath bombs rejuvenate you and make your skin smooth and supple. Moreover, you have a bath bomb for every occasion! Since they are so beautiful and dainty looking, they also make perfect gifts for loved ones.

This book is a guide for bath bombs, and the various question you may have regarding them. This book also has many great recipes that will push you to create beautiful and creative bath bombs within a very defined budget. So, experiment a bit and make some awesome creations. Gift them, keep them, enjoy them. Remember, this is something that helps you pamper yourself and recognize you own worth.

Go ahead. Put on some music, throw in a bath bomb, dive in the bathtub and experience your homemade first-class spa!

FROM THE AUTHOR

I would like to ask you for a small favor. If you have a minute, please leave a comment under my book.

Thank You!

Check Out My Other Books

Bellow you will find my other books that are popular on Amazon.

Health & beauty:

Body Scrubs: 30 Organic Homemade Body And Face Scrubs, The Best All-Natural Recipes For Soft, Radiant And Youthful Skin

Natural Hair Care Guide: How To Stop Hair Loss And Accelerate Hair Growth In A Natural Way, Get Strong, Healthy And Shiny Hair Without Chemicals

Essential Oils Guide: The Ultimate Guide To Essential Oils For Weight Loss, Stress Relief, Aromatherapy, Beauty Care, Easy Recipes For Health & Beauty

Essential Oils For Pets: Essential Oils For Dogs: 40 Safe & Effective Therapies And Remedies To Keep Your Dog Healthy From Puppy To Adult

Essential Oils For Cats: Safe & Effective Therapies And Remedies To Keep Your Cat Healthy And Happy

Anti-Aging Skin Care Secrets: Younger Skin Without Scalpel And Botox. Discover How To Rejuvenate Your Skin Quickly And Maintain A Youthful Appearance

Growing orchids:

Orchids: Growing Orchids Made Easy And Pleasant. The Most Common Errors In The Cultivation Of Orchids. Let Your Orchids Grow For Many Years

Phalaenopsis Orchids Care: 30 Most Important Things To Remember When Growing Phalaenopsis Orchids, How To Give The Best Life To Your Plants

Orchids Care For Hobbyists: The Advanced Guide For Orchid Enthusiasts

Orchids Care Bundle (Orchids + Orchids Care For Hobbyists): Growing Orchids Made Easy And Pleasant + The Advanced Guide For Orchid Enthusiasts

Phalaenopsis Orchids Box Set 2 in 1: Phalaenopsis Orchids Care + Orchids Care For Hobbyists

Orchids Care Bundle 3 in 1: Orchids + Orchids Care For Hobbyists + Phalaenopsis Orchids Care

Speed Reading Guide For Beginners:

Speed Reading Guide For Beginners: Get Your Fast Reading Skill The Easy Way. Simple Techniques To Increase Your Reading Speed In Less 24 Hours

You can simply search for the titles on the Amazon website to find them.

Best regards!

Made in the USA
San Bernardino, CA
18 February 2017